The Secrets to Healthy Aging: Reverse the Signs of Aging at Any Age

Dedication

When The Dalai Lama was asked what surprised him most he said, "Man. Because he sacrifices his health in order to make money. Then he sacrifices money to recuperate his health."

In order to change your body and your health you must first change your mind. This guide is your roadmap to restoring youth, creasting lasting health, and regaining authority and control over how you will age. Read It, Learn It and then Live It. Enjoy the Journey!

~ Coach Nikole

The Secrets to Healthy Aging: Reverse the Signs of Aging at Any Age

Nikole Seals

Nourished Minds

PUBLICATIONS
2014

First Printing: 2014

ISBN 13: 978-0-9915063-0-9

Published and distributed in the Unites States by Nourished Minds

www.NourishedMinds.com

Contents

Chapter 1: My Story

"There is one consolation to being sick; and
that is the possibility that you may recover to a
better state than you were ever in before."
~ Henry David Thoreau

I have never spent the night in a hospital and I
can count the number of times I've been in the
emergency room on one hand. So it was difficult
for me to understand, how at the age of 31, I found
myself dressed only in my underwear, haphazardly
covered with a hospital gown, undergoing an
electrocardiogram (EKG). I had driven myself to
the ER after convincing my client not to call for an
ambulance. You see, I had been in the middle of a
therapy session when I was afflicted by a series of
severe chest pains. The pains originated near the
center of my ribcage and would then ripple
throughout my body in the form of a dull ache.
However, they came and went like contractions so
I had figured that I had a fifteen minute window to
get myself to a hospital.

During that ten minute drive, I kept asking
myself why this was happening. I had been healthy
and active as a young adult and was in great shape
for a woman in her early thirties. I was working out
more than ever and had just completed a month on
the South Beach diet that resulted in me dropping
ten pounds. Sure, work had been incredibly
stressful and as a result, I sometimes resorted to
eating fast food on those nights when I worked

late. But I figured that wouldn't be enough to send me into cardiac arrest.

By the time I got to the hospital, the pain was so bad that I could barely talk and breathing had become difficult. I will say this, walking into the ER dripping in sweat and clutching your chest is a sure fire way to bypass the waiting room. They took me in immediately and prepared me for the EKG. When the nurse went to place the adhesive disc on my chest, I yelped out in pain. My entire ribcage felt like it was on fire! I was extremely tender to the touch and bless her heart; she used such care and apologized with each one of those sticky things she put on me.

The doctor had not been as empathetic. He poked and tapped and pressed to the point that I had to ask him to stop. He inquired if I had any other unusual symptoms that he should know about. With limited breath, I reported the strange and random symptoms I had been experiencing over the past year. Like the re-occurring rashes that would appear on my legs and arms that burned and often left scars. There were also the pains I would get in my joints that I just attributed to aging or over doing it at the gym. And then there were the digestive problems. As if laying on the hospital bed with all my goods on display wasn't embarrassing enough, I told the doctor how things weren't running so smoothly with my stomach. I mentioned the severe cramping that I would sometimes experience in the middle of the night. He wrote it all down and told me to try and get some rest while we waited for my test results.

A few hours had passed and I had started feeling better but I'm certain that was because of the pain medication they gave me. Thankfully, it also helped to numb me to the persistent moaning of a fellow patient and the controlled chaos that seemed to come rushing through the ER doors every 20 minutes.

My final prognosis: Costochondritis, or in layman's terms, inflammation of the chest wall. Basically the muscles in my chest were inflamed and they were constricting my lungs, which is why I felt the tightness. He prescribed me a bout of steroids and an anti-inflammatory. When I had asked what caused it, he told me that most often it's stress or anxiety. But he never really explained the how or why. And he most certainly did not give me any helpful tips on resolving the problem. I already knew my job was a great source of stress in my life but what was I supposed to do...quit?

His answer was that I try taking anti-anxiety medication. I declined. As a therapist, I understood that stress was a normal reaction and unavoidable at times and didn't want to have to rely on medication to cope with it. I would do it the old fashion way...ignore it.

As for my other symptoms, the doctor didn't have a clue. He said that they might be related to the stress or some other "underlying medical condition". He didn't seem to have any interest in clearing up the mystery and sent me away with a goodie bag of medications.

The steroids made me gain weight. With ease, I put back on the ten pounds I had lost and then some. Two months later, the chest pains were back and brought a friend along with them: joint pains. I had pain in places that I didn't even know I had joints. Even my knuckles ached. Writing and typing for work had become difficult and working out only happened on the days that I could take a deep breath without wincing in pain.

Over the next two years, my health declined significantly. I masked what was going on for as long as I could because I didn't want to worry my family. I kept working yet started a journal of my symptoms. I went from seeing a doctor once a year for my annual check-up to a visit every other month. The frequency of my pain increased as did my rashes. I was diagnosed with anemia, migraines, fibromyalgia and irritable bowel syndrome for which I got a new goodie bag of meds. Oh, and did I mention that I had started getting cortisone shots in my legs to deal with the pain? My life carried on this way until two very profound things happened to me.

The first was when I realized that my repeated use of steroids had changed my appetite and caused me to have insomnia. I started craving carbohydrates and was emotionally eating on a regular basis. But it was the lack of sleep that started pushing me over the edge. I was cranky, frustrated and depressed.

I went to see a highly recommended doctor and took all of my journal notes and old prescriptions, hoping that he would finally be able to fix me. I remember how he glanced at my empty prescription bottles and didn't even bother to read my notes. Actually, he showed very little interest in what had occurred in my life prior to the moment I walked in his office.

This doctor spent a total of fifteen minutes with me before he diagnosed me with depression. He told me that my situation was very common in women and that many, if not all of my symptoms, were brought on by my depression. He scribbled out a prescription for Prozac. I took it, crumbled it up, and told him to go to Hell. Maybe it was the sleep deprivation or my alleged depression talking but I was officially done playing the guessing game.

The final crushing blow came three weeks later when a teenager that I was interviewing for work asked me if I had grandchildren. Out of the mouths of babes, right? But this wasn't an innocent kindergartner; this was a 17 year-old young man who had just noticed what I had been refusing to notice.

That night, I went home and pulled out photos of myself from two years ago and was stunned. I had aged. In just two years I went from looking five years younger than my actual age to looking five years older than my actual age. That's ten years! Upon careful examination in the mirror, I had also noticed that I had way more gray hairs than I use to. Then I felt it; a patch of baldness, right on the crown of my head. It was about the size of a vanilla wafer cookie. I sobbed uncontrollably. But to this day, I'm so very glad it happened. Because that is the moment I took back control of my mind and body.

I started to read everything I could about health and nutrition. That's how I learned about the practice of naturopathic medicine. Naturopathic medicine looks to treat patients by restoring overall health instead of suppressing a few key symptoms with medication. Practitioners seek to find the underlying causes of the symptoms and develop treatment plans that utilize the body's own natural healing mechanisms. It is based on five principles of healing.

1. Nature before technology – meaning that practitioners look to use the least invasive methods possible, especially those found in nature

2. Focus is centered on the patient, rather than the physician – that is that a physician should look to learn as much as he/she can from a patient rather than focusing on all that he has learned in med school; the bottom line is that a patient's history is a critical part of care

3. First, do no harm – physicians should really try to avoid causing unnecessary harm to a patient; for example, performing a C-section

just for scheduling convenience or prescribing the wrong medications

4. Results take longer – meaning that naturopathic medicine doesn't buy into the theory of a "magic pill" to fix everything and rather tries to stimulate the body's natural abilities to heal itself

5. Promotes the use of purely natural substances – this type of alternative medicine is open to using natural substances from all over the world that have been in use for thousands of years and proven to be effective

Listen, I don't want you thinking that I'm not a fan of conventional medicine because I am. What I can't support is the decline in care that has become a common characteristic of our healthcare system. I didn't want to medicate my body, I wanted to heal it. But in the span of those few years, I believe that the medical intervention I had received was actually a contributing factor in the accelerated aging of my body. And when you are still young in the mind but living in an aged body, you are living out of balance. And that imbalance affects your mind and your emotions. That was unacceptable to me.

So I went and saw a naturopathic physician. I will never forget that first visit; mainly because it lasted an entire hour! She took copious notes on everything I said and even made copies of pages from my journal to keep on record. Now that I look back on it, I think she knew what my problem was on day one but she wanted to run some test to be thorough. And boy was she thorough. She sent me on my way with lab orders for a series of test (I mention these in details later in the guide); nothing too invasive but some I had never even heard of, let alone did I know what they would reveal.

Three weeks later I was back in her office for my results. The diagnosis was toxicity, sometimes referred to as autointoxication. To put it bluntly, I was filled with a bunch of yeast, toxic chemicals, and crap. I was floored, but what was more astonishing was her explanation as to how I became toxic. One of the test revealed that I was allergic to peanuts. It was a mild allergy that went unnoticed because my reaction was mainly happening internally. See my body, for whatever reason, has a difficult time processing the amino acid arguinine, which is found in high concentrations in peanuts. This makes quite a bit of sense seeing as I have been allergic to chocolate my entire life and chocolate is also high in arguinine.

Now, do you remember when I told you that I started having symptoms about one month after I had been on the South Beach Diet? Well, while I was on that diet, I consumed peanut butter on a daily basis. Here I was thinking I was being healthy while in reality, I was making myself very sick. This is not to criticize the South Beach Diet but to point out how important it is that you become proactive in getting to know your body and manage its care.

There were several other factors that were causing my toxicity, which is basically the process of self-poisoning caused by bacteria, waste, and other poisons being produced within the body.

Because of my high-stress job, I continually had high levels of the stress hormone cortisol (I'll explain in chapter two how this hormone impacts the health of our bodies)

I was dehydrated (most of us are...you'll find out exactly how much water you should be drinking later in this guide)

I had an overgrowth of bacteria in my digestive tract and as a result, my colon was struggling to absorb nutrients from my food and eliminate waste (the reason for my constipation and cramping)

When I made poor food choices, I deprived my body of vital nutrients and as a result I had several nutritional deficiencies

For the purpose of this guide, it is important that you understand how all of these things increased the speed at which my body was aging. I will go more into detail as we progress through this guide but the premise of it all boils down to two things: nourishment and regeneration. Think of a plant...if you don't feed it properly and maintain it, it will wither and eventually die. The same is true for our bodies. The body needs proper nourishment to regenerate or grow new cells. If you are sick, toxic, and depriving your body of nutrients, it can only grow sick unhealthy new cells to replace the sick unhealthy old ones. But when you are in a state of health and giving your body the tools it needs in the form of nutrient dense foods, it can grown healthy new cells to replace the old ones.

I know this to be true because that is exactly what happened for me. With the help of my naturopathic physician, I took back control of my body. It didn't happen overnight and it took some work but the results have been amazing.

I stopped having symptoms about three months after my first visit with the naturopathic physician. It has been over ten years and I have never had a need for any of the medications I use to take daily. I am back to visiting the doctor just once a year for my annual check-up. I still catch a cold once every blue moon but my body has learned how to heal itself and so I require no medical intervention. I sleep like a baby and weigh the same as I did when I was in college...for my undergraduate degree.

The best part of this story is that I have never looked better. No one can guess my age and I've even had people ask in disbelief to see my driver's license. I stopped having rashes, my skin is clear and glowing, and I no longer have to dye my hair to cover the gray. It just goes to show you how the right information can change your life.

I share this story about the most difficult time of my life because I know that I'm not the only person to have had such an experience. I'm just one of many who have learned how to help my body naturally heal itself. I know *The Secrets to Healthy Aging* will work for you if you apply them to your life because they have worked for me and many of my clients. With the right information found in this guide, you can learn how to help your body instead of harming it and *Reverse the Signs of Aging at Any Age.*

Chapter 2: Investing in Your Health

Yes, the Fountain of Youth is real and you don't have to travel to an exotic location to find it. As a matter of fact, it's as easy as walking into your kitchen and opening up the refrigerator. Wah-La! It's all right there. Well, maybe not right this minute but after you read this book you will be armed with all the knowledge you need to slow the aging process and look and feel your best.

From this moment on, you are no longer thinking of aging as the process where you get old, have less energy and idly sit by and watch everything go to Hell in a hand basket. You accept that it is a natural process that every living thing must go through. However, you now know that you have the power to determine if you are going to age slowly and enjoy a life full of vitality and good health or if you are going to do things that may actually age you faster than time itself.

I am a firm believer that the human body was designed to maintain its full capabilities and balance as we age. The reason we don't see this happening is because of man's free will. The food choices we make, the environmental factors we expose ourselves to, even the careers and people we choose to have in our lives all play a role in how we age. But the best part of having free will is that at any time in our lives we can choose to live in a way that slows down aging and helps us to retain some of our youthful characteristics. And I imagine that if I have kept your interest thus far, it's because you no longer want to race to the finish line of old age. Why not get there at a nice casual pace that allows you to experience life while looking and feeling your best?

This book is for adults of all ages because unfortunately, many of our poor dietary habits start when we are teens and set us on a course for accelerated aging long before we open our first 401K. We've all met the twenty-something who really looked thirty-something or know of someone who has struggled with an illness and watched them age right before our eyes. Everyone can benefit from this guide, even if they are currently healthy and in great shape. Because it's not just about healthy aging; our ultimate goal is to prolong the state of youthfulness. Don't you want your so called golden years to be free of pain, disability, illness and a dependence on others for your care?

Speaking of which, did you know that the population of retirees in America is exploding at this very moment? As you read, legions of baby boomers are starting to leave the work force and its having a tremendous impact on our healthcare system, as well as our social security system. The cost of medical care is on the rise and some seniors are finding that the majority of their monthly social security income is needed to cover the cost of medication, treatment and in-home care. We also tend to live in a society that would rather medicate you than educate you. The sad truth is that if you are a baby boomer, you can't afford to get sick unless you have a considerable nest egg set aside. Or you can choose to make an investment in your health today so that you're not paying for it tomorrow.

The *Secrets to Healthy Aging* aren't really secrets because the fact is that these simple tips have been practiced by people all over the world; all throughout history. I refer to them as secrets because industries like Pharmaceuticals, Tobacco, Dairy, Medical, and especially the Food industry, don't want you to learn how to properly care for and nourish your body. If you get healthy, who would pay the high insurance premiums, or become dependent on medications, or purchase their products that provide you with no health benefits whatsoever? They would go out of business. That's why you see more commercials for Lipitor than you do for flaxseed.

The secrets that I am about to share with you have nothing to do with diets, fads, gimmicks, trends, or the latest in cosmetology science. You don't need to spend a lot of money to slow the aging process. And you most definitely don't need to do anything drastic like surgery or having someone inject a toxin into your face. A healthy glow and vitality start from within.

The *Secrets to Healthy Aging* are simple things that you can incorporate into your lifestyle in order to prevent your body from aging faster than it should. These steps are natural in that they do not involve the use of any chemicals or medication; only essential nutrients and easy to find supplements. The only cost that you will incur is in the purchase of this book and in the purchase of quality versions of things you already buy, like food.

The most important of these practices are the ones that will teach you how to avoid the things that cause your body to age at an accelerated rate. Excessive wrinkles, damaged skin, aching joints, chronic illness, disease; all of it is avoidable. Learn how to feel better, live longer, and look good doing it.

This book was written to be used as a quick reference or guide on what you can do today to *Reverse the Signs of Aging at Any Age*. It is intentionally devoid of all the fluff and repetition you would find in most health books. The science behind nutrition and aging is complicated but I will make it easy by teaching you exactly *what* you need to do and *why* so that you can determine the best way to incorporate these practices into your life.

Healthcare vs. Preventative Care

Our healthcare system in the U.S. is in a state of crisis.

The Congressional Budget Office determined that in 2009, we spent more per capitia on healthcare than any other nation in the world.

Yet the World Health Organization (WHO) rated the US 37ᵗʰ (out of 40 nations!) in our ability to treat and care for patients.

According to the U.S. Census Bureau, between 2000 and 2010, the population of 45 to 64 years old grew 31.5 percent to 81.5 million, making it 26.4 percent of the total US population.

When people think of aging, they often visualize a life of doctor visits, nursing homes and a bedside nightstand littered with prescription bottles. Unfortunately, this has become the reality for many people, some of which have yet to even reach retirement age. But it's not the passing of time that is stealing our youth; it's us. We are the culprits—well, us and our partners in crime: the Food and Drug Industries.

Americans have become mass consumers of processed foods and the food industry is much obliged to provide us with a never ending supply of food (and I use that term loosely) that is basically devoid of nutrients. The problem is that our bodies can't utilize the ingredients in such foods and often these same ingredients are hazardous to our health. So in the process of filling our bodies with harmful chemicals, additives, dyes, and over processed grains, we deprive it of the nutrients it needs to thrive.

If you wanted to build a house that would shelter and protect you for many, many years to come, would you build it out of plywood and toxic glue? Do you think the Egyptian pyramids would still be standing if the contractor decided to go on the cheap and use sand instead of stone? The reality is that if you want something to last, you use the best quality materials you can find. And in the case of making our bodies time proof, we need to be eating nutrient dense foods that help us to replenish, repair and rebuild. If you are in it for the long haul, then you must begin choosing foods that will help you to stand the test of time.

When it comes to modern medicine, we must first acknowledge the amazing advances in the field of science that are responsible for saving people's lives. Medicine is essential and vitally important to our health; especially when we talk about emergency medicine. The fact is that if you get hit by a car and get rushed into the emergency room, you don't want the doctor to tell you to eat some broccoli while he dabs tree tea oil on your wounds. You want the fast acting, potent stuff that's going to keep you from bleeding out or stop you from getting a life threatening infection.

The problem is that medicine has become so good at being a "quick fix" that we turn to it for virtually any ailment or symptom that we have. Have a cough? Take some cough syrup. Gassy from that late night double cheeseburger? Take an antacid. Can't sleep? No problem, take a sleeping pill.

Americans love the fast acting effects of drugs. So much so that some pharmaceutical CEO's are making in estimate of 22 million dollars a year in salary plus an additional 250 million in stock options. A healthy you puts them out of business but a sick you keeps them rolling in the green. It's a win/win for the drug industry if they can convince you that you need to be on blood pressure medication for the remainder of your life. You become dependent and they get you as a lifetime customer without the hassle of having to do any customer service or quality control. And if you think medications are expensive now, just wait and see what happens to the prices over the next 10-20 years.

If this guide helps you to do anything, the hope is that it enables you to never have to be dependent on medications and to keep you out of the hospital. Again, hospitals are the place you want to be in the case of an emergency but otherwise, try to stay out of them. Even the *American Journal of Medicine* acknowledges the high rate of deaths that are a result of unnecessary surgeries, medication errors, negative effects of drugs and hospital caused infections. You could go in with a broken leg and come out with something entirely different and possibly more life threatening. You might go in for chest pains and come out with a staph infection and an exorbitant bill on top of it.

The Department of Commerce has noted the average prescription cost at $70; a visit to the emergency room for the cost of $700 and treatment for an acute incident like a heart attack in upwards of $45,000 to $50,000. (Note these are averages and can differ based on the state where you live and the type of insurance you have)

Now if the broken leg, staph infection and the bill don't kill you, then it's always possible that the hospital food might. Okay, it won't actually kill you but it won't actually help. For anyone who has eaten hospital food, you know what I mean. Hospital meal plans are largely based on the recommendations of the USDA and the standard American diet (SAD). So the menu often resembles the recently retired food pyramid that has governed our hospital meals and school lunches for far too long. It is completely self defeating but hospitals tend to serve the worst kind and the worst quality of foods.

I once had a client go into the emergency room for atrial fibrillation (irregular heartbeat) during the last trimester of her pregnancy. When I showed up to visit her, she was eating a grilled cheese sandwich. Now if someone was presenting with symptoms that are also risk factors of cardiovascular disease, it just seems like good sense to veto the cheesy sandwich and give the patient foods rich in magnesium, calcium, potassium, vitamin C and essential fatty acids.

These vital nutrients are important for proper cardiac muscle function and for regulating blood pressure and can be found in foods like leafy greens, fruits, cold water fish, nuts, and avocados. And let's add to that list the amino acid Taurine (found in high protein foods) which has been proven to help stabilize the heartbeat and correct arrhythmias. You may find it interesting to know that heart healthy diets often recommend avoiding foods like white bread, butter, fried foods and hydrogenated oils; the very components of a grilled cheese sandwich!

Yes, hospitals save lives but they also focus on treatment, not prevention and nutrition which is where the healthcare industry's focus should be. The good news is that if you're reading this guidebook, you're already ahead of the game and well on your way to experiencing a drug and hospital free life.

The reality is that we all want to look our best and retain some aspects of our youth, like healthy skin, good teeth, an alert mind and a body that allows us to engage in the physical activities we enjoy. And I, along with countless other professionals in the field of nutrition, holistic health and alternative medicine, believe that good health can be enjoyed well into your eighties and nineties. That's because the body was designed to naturally regenerate itself continuously throughout our lifetime. That's right. Every few years we get a new body. Our cells are constantly dying and regenerating to form new hair, new skin, new tissue, and so on. The problem is that we are also introducing new factors into our lives and diets that damage these cells and our DNA, resulting in inflammation, illness and disease.

Would you believe me if I told you that by simply making a few changes to your lifestyle and the foods you eat, you could look and feel younger, minimize the need for medical intervention and live longer? Would that convince you to make the investment in your health today? It should. And if you mindfully read through this book and adopt these secret tips into your life that is exactly what will happen. It's time to take the fear out of aging and put the focus back on living.

Chapter 3: Nutrient Thieves:
Stealing Your Youth

The first and I believe most important step in slowing the aging process is to avoid or eliminate those things in your life that deplete your body of precious nutrients. Nutrients are the essence of life; they are capable of growing life and sustaining life. Without them you would die. And when they are scarce in our bodies or destroyed by other substances, we become ill and susceptible to disease.

All of the changes that we see occurring in our bodies and write off as the aging process are actually signs from the body that it is in a nutrient deficient state. Many people just accept these changes and or succumb to disease with the mindset that it's due to genetics. And yes, our DNA does play a role. Recent studies have revealed that our DNA is affected by not only environmental factors but also by the foods we eat. Nutritional deficiencies and high levels of toxins can alter or trigger certain genetic traits. For an example, if you have a family history of heart attacks, you increase your risk and may possibly trigger that gene if you smoke or eat a diet high in fatty foods. If you don't smoke, eat healthy, and exercise; that gene may never be triggered and you may never have a heart attack.

In this section, we'll focus on those things that you consume or expose yourself to that are depleting nutrients in your body. Here is my list of the Top Six Nutrient Killers that you need to avoid if at all possible.

1. SUGAR

Yes, I know this one is hard to hear but I made it number one for a reason. There are countless studies that have proven how sugar accelerates the aging process. It will age you faster than time, and unfortunately, Americans are consuming it in large quantities. According to the U.S. Department of Agriculture, the average American consumes 150 pounds of sugar a year or roughly, the equivalent of 52 teaspoons a day (the USDA recommends no more than 6 tsp per day). This is the reason behind the obesity epidemic in this country in both adults and children.

So how exactly is this deliciously sweet substance harmful to your body? Well for starters, and probably most important is that sugar hinders the body's immune system from functioning properly. It alters the quantity and activity of white blood cells. And when your immune system is suppressed, you are more susceptible to illness and disease.

An equally important consequence to eating sugar is the fact that it has a severe effect your blood glucose levels. All of us have experienced a "sugar high" and the, "I just need to rest my head on my desk for a minute" low that quickly follows.

Once that simple sugar is converted into energy and used, we experience the withdrawal effect and then we crave more sugar to wake us up. Meanwhile, our body is constantly producing insulin in order to regulate the sugar in our bloodstream and balance out the highs and lows. Years of this cycle strains the body's ability to produce insulin and the next thing you know, your doctor is diagnosing you with diabetes. And all that excess sugar that your body couldn't handle and converted to fat has propelled you into the weight class of obese.

But wait, that's not all; add to that the use of artificial sweeteners like Aspartame (found in Equal, and NutraSweet) and you increase your risk of cancer, heart disease, digestive disorders, mood disorders, sleep disorders, and overall body toxicity. Both sugar and the chemicals in artificial sweeteners can damage the health of your arteries, alter hormonal balance, impair tissue growth and cause a whole host of health conditions. And if you check with the Food and Drug Administration, you may be surprised to find out that Aspartame has caused 75% of all adverse food reactions reported in recent years. Still sound delicious? The thing is that it is unrealistic to try to remove all sugar from your diet but you can add years to your life by greatly reducing how much sugar you eat and avoiding harmful sweeteners.

2. PROCESSED FOODS AND FOOD CHEMICALS

I am always confounded when I read labels on food packages or hear advertisements that claim "enriched with vitamins". Let's talk about what that really means.

Basically, a food manufacturer takes a natural food like wheat in its whole grain form and processes it into a fine powder, what we refer to as wheat flour. What happens during "processing" is that the wheat grain gets stripped of its coating, fibrous content, proteins and essential oils, to the extent that is loses much of its natural nutrients. Even worst is that they often use chemicals to bleach this powder to produce white flour!

The manufacturer now has flour that can be used in thousands of different food products but really offers no nutritional value. So what do they do? They add synthetic vitamins and minerals to the flour and call it "enriched". The problem is that it is difficult for the human body to absorb synthetic vitamins and minerals unlike naturally occurring nutrients that are easily recognized by the body. So when you eat highly processed foods, you are essentially eating food with little or no nutritional value or what I call "dead foods". These foods also contain hidden sugar (by using cleverly deceptive wording), salts and fats. A good rule of thumb is to avoid all enriched flour products; choose breads and pastas made with whole grains; and choose baked foods over fried.

Processed food is loaded with chemicals like additives, dyes, preservatives and flavoring, while fruits and vegetables are tainted with chemicals like pesticides. And if that wasn't enough, biogenetic food scientists have created genetically modified foods (GMOs) to further complicate our pursuit of quality foods.

Why would we intentionally contaminate our food? Well, manufacturers were tickled at the idea that they could increase the shelf life of a food or allegedly enhance its flavor and appearance by adding chemicals. No one was too concerned about the long term effects of this experiment until studies started to reveal the link between consumption of these chemicals and health conditions like allergies, skin abnormalities, infertility, depression, migraines and memory decline. The problem is that we don't just consume these chemicals and then eliminate them in our waste. They actually get stored in our cells...for a very, very long time. Don't believe me? Ever wonder how people can be drug tested for past substance use with a hair follicle test? These toxic substances don't disappear; they stay in us and cause us great harm.

Genetically modified foods go so far as to insert other plant, animal and human DNA into foods to make them, "super foods". The goal is to create a new species of food (that agricultural companies patent and own, of course) that is indestructible to viruses and bacteria with its own internal pesticide to protect it. This is not a new science. In fact there are already many forms of GMO foods on the market today such as soy, corn and sugar beets. And as of yet, the government is not requiring these foods to be labeled so you really have no idea when they will show up on your plate.

You can avoid these chemicals and altered foods by purchasing organic products whenever possible. It may cost a little bit more so stick to purchasing those fruits and vegetables that are known to have high levels of pesticide residue, *aka* "The Dirty Dozen". They include: peaches, apples, bell peppers, celery, lettuce, pears, nectarines, spinach, cherries, grapes, strawberries, and potatoes. You'll be fine buying regular commercial versions of produce with thick outer skins like bananas, avocadoes, cantaloupes and oranges. If you can't afford the additional cost or don't live in an area that offers organic versions, then try to purchase from small local farmers or get your produce from friends, family or neighbors who have fruit trees and gardens. Better yet, grow your own!

3. STRESS

This nutrient killer can easily share the number one spot as it has a profound effect on the body. First, you must understand what happens when we experience a stressful thought or situation. The body responds to stress by releasing the stress hormones adrenaline and cortisol. These hormones prepare the body for what has been termed the fight-or-flight syndrome. This occurs when the body creates a surge of energy to fuel itself for a battle or quick escape (for example, moving out of the way of an oncoming car). Our heart rate increases, blood pressure increases, muscles contract and the body continues to searches for more energy. When this state of stress is prolonged, the body eventually depletes its resources and enters into a stage of exhaustion.

The most important thing to know about this process is that it doesn't matter what type of stress you experience; the body reacts the same, whether it's emotional, physical, mental, or chemical. It doesn't matter if it's from a car accident, giving a speech, watching a scary movie, having an argument, losing your car keys, or walking into your surprise birthday party. It all registers the same.

However, the body was not designed to be in a chronic state of stress and what eventually happens is a domino effect with our body systems. Damage occurs to our adrenal and thymus glands, the immune system gets overwhelmed, toxins and bacteria grow without regulation, food does not get digested properly and nutrients don't get absorbed or get depleted. The management of stress requires magnesium to be pulled from our cells, calcium to be stolen from our bones and depletes the body of the very necessary B vitamins.

According to a 2007 study by the American Psychological Association, 1 out of 5 respondents reached their highest stress level 15 or more days per month while 77% said that they had experienced physical problems due to their stress.

Stress that goes unmanaged can cause all kinds of symptoms and disease: chest pain, cancer, constipation, eczema, high blood pressure, irritable bowel syndrome, joint pain, neck and back pain, ulcers, PMS, psoriasis, sexual problems and weight loss/gain just to name a few.

Groundbreaking research conducted in 2004 at the University of San Francisco, by Blackburn and Epel found that stress accelerated the aging process by damaging the DNA that controls cell aging. Meaning that unmanaged stress actually has the ability to speed up the rate at which your cells age!

So, how do you eliminate stress from your life? Well you can't. But you can limit your exposure to it and control how you react to it. We'll discuss how further along in the book but for now...don't stress over it.

4.   ENVIRONMENTAL TOXINS

They're everywhere and more often than not, hidden from plain view. They are the invisible nutrient-killers and the most difficult to avoid. They include toxic cleaning products, pesticides, radiation, heavy metals in our water supply, tobacco smoke, chemicals in our plastics, and pollutants in the air.

These toxins, some of which are carcinogens, enter into our bodies by mouth and skin and form what are known as free radicals. They are termed free radicals because they are molecules that are capable of existing on their own yet will attack other healthy cells in the body. It is believed that signs and symptoms of aging are in fact the breakdown of these attacked cells. To limit your exposure, try to avoid using harsh chemicals: instead, clean your home with regular soap, vinegar, baking soda and rubbing alcohol. Also avoid all tobacco smoke and the use of pesticides inside or outside of your home. Later, I will discuss how to choose quality drinking water.

5. BEVERAGES

I use this all inclusive title because there are several forms of beverages that you need to limit or avoid in the pursuit of health. They are soda, caffeinated beverages and alcohol. I know, I know. You like to have a glass of wine with dinner or need to start your day with a cup of Joe. I am not suggesting that you completely eliminate these beverages from your diet, but I do want you to know how they affect your health and the speed at which you are aging.

Let's start with soda. Soda is the fifth-largest source of calories for adults. It has no nutritional value and fills you up with sugar, additives and caffeine. More importantly, people choose it over drinking water so the body becomes dehydrated. Soft drink consumption has been linked to obesity, tooth decay, heart disease, kidney stones and gout.

Remember when we talked about trying to balance blood sugar levels and how sugars offset this balance? Well caffeine has a very similar effect on the body. You may be surprised to learn that caffeine is not what gives you energy. It stimulates the release of stored glucose into the bloodstream and that is actually where the boost of energy comes from; not from caffeine. When you think about it, caffeine is basically tricking your body. See the body reacts to stimulants just as if it had consumed food. It secretes insulin to regulate your blood sugar level and since you didn't actually eat anything, there is nothing to replenish your energy stores. That's why the coffee high never seems to last very long and has you feeling like you need more.

Caffeine also prevents the absorption of vital minerals like calcium, magnesium, iron, zinc, selenium, chromium. I should also mention that as we age, we produce less acid/digestive enzymes so we really can't afford to exacerbate the problem by drinking excessive amounts of caffeinated beverages. Limit it to one 12 oz serving per day, preferably in the morning when it will promote the elimination of waste. Or try drinking a healthy version of your favorite beverage that has little or no caffeine like herbal teas.

The least favorite suggestion that I make to my clients is to limit their intake of alcohol. They usually respond by rolling their eyes or giving me a blank stare. Some have just outright told me, "No". And I always say, "Your body, your choice." But then I remind them that they can't complain about the appearance of their skin, the weight gain, or the difficulties they have sleeping; all of which can be directly related to alcohol consumption. My recommendation is that if you really like your cocktails, then at least try to drink in moderation and detoxify/cleanse your liver and digestive tract on a regular basis. If you want the pleasure of drinking alcohol than you must do the required damage repair.

Alcohol is taxing on your liver and prevents the absorption of important B vitamins. Alcohol is also dehydrating and pulls water away from other necessary body functions. What many people are surprised to learn is that alcohol converts to sugar in your body and we've already discussed the harmful effects of sugar. Excessive alcohol in your body will accelerate the overgrowth of yeast in your digestive tract. This yeast is responsible for conditions such as constipation, diarrhea, irritable bowel syndrome (IBS), bladder infections, kidney infections, vaginal yeast infections, body odor, skin problems, migraines, and many more.

If you know someone who struggles with alcoholism, then chances are you have seen how alcohol can age people well beyond their years. In addition, alcohol is very disruptive to the body's natural sleep patterns. It may help you to relax and fall asleep but it can actually cause you to wake up during the night or prevent you from having good deep sleep. As you'll learn later on in this guidebook, sleep is instrumental in rejuvenating the body and slowing the aging process.

6. HOMOCYSTEINE

You don't hear much about homocysteine from doctors or in the news but it is one of the best indicators as to your current and future state of health. Here are the basics that you need to know about homocysteine: it is a type of amino acid that is produced in the body and found in the blood; under normal circumstances the body is able to manufacture this amino acid into other helpful substances in the body; too much homocysteine in your blood is an indicator that you are at an increased risk for over fifty diseases.

So what causes homocysteine to go from a manageable, helpful level to one that can cause serious harm? In his book, *Age-Defying Diet Revolution*, Dr. Atkins explains that homocysteine increases not as a result of what you eat but as a result of what you *don't* eat. He states that "elevated homocysteine is a result of vitamin deficiency" and that it "may be one of the direct causes of aging itself." That's because the body needs an adequate supply of B vitamins in order to make the enzyme that removes homocysteine from the blood and converts it into beneficial substances.

Recent studies are finding that high levels of homocysteine in the blood can damage your arteries, brain, and your cell DNA. One of the best ways to manage this protein is to regularly consume foods rich in B vitamins (especially folic acid) and avoid those things that will deplete vitamins in your body. Remember, stress, alcohol, caffeine, and environmental toxins will deplete or prevent the absorption of B vitamins, resulting in elevated levels of homocysteine.

Hopefully you are starting to realize that avoiding certain things in your diet and lifestyle is just as important as choosing quality nutrient rich foods. Now that we have discussed many of the villains that will rob you of your youth, let's turn our focus to the foods and nutritional supplements that will not only aid you in maintaining good health but can help you to look and feel your best.

Chapter 4: Your Anti-Aging Hero

Chances are that during the time you have been reading this book, you've either had a snack, experienced hunger, or you were thinking about your next meal. Maybe you've been sipping on a refreshing glass of iced tea while taking note of the ways in which you may be unknowingly aging yourself. That's the whole point: to get you thinking about what you put in your body.

Now, I want you to take a moment and think about your next meal. Even if you are in your pajamas and all cozy in your bed, take a minute and think about what you are going to have for breakfast. Close your eyes and visualize that meal in your head. Is it just one type of food or does your meal consists of a mixture of several food types? Now ask yourself, what is that food(s) going to do for my body? Is it going to nourish my body or is it going to be harmful to my body?

Keep in mind that if you are eating foods that have no nutritional value, they are causing more harm than good. That's because processed foods require energy, water, nutrients, and enzymes in order to be broken down in your digestive tract. Your body goes through great effort to digest it and gets nothing in return. We want to eat foods that give us more energy than it requires.

Next I want you to ask yourself, why am I eating this particular food? Are you eating it for nourishment or for pleasure? Are you eating with a health purpose in mind or to satisfy an urge or feeling? I'll bet many of you will be surprised to find that the majority of your food choices are mostly made for pleasure.

When you think about the quality of your foods and the nutritional content, you gain some insight into why you choose certain foods. For example, if you visualized eating a bagel with gobs of cream cheese in the morning, then you my friend are eating for pleasure. Your choice is made based on your habitual thoughts and cravings rather than with a purpose. I call this type of decision making—emotional eating.

Emotional eating is when your feelings are making food choices for you; like if you've had a particularly bad day and you find yourself eating a pint of ice cream. Or say you are stressed and running late, so you decide to grab a muffin at Starbucks to go with your 600 calorie coffee. I see this behavior in many of my clients and remember, I have had my own personal experience with emotional eating.

During the days when I was counseling families in crisis, I experienced a high level of stress and frustration on a daily basis. That ongoing stress had me seeking all kinds of comfort foods; pizza, French fries, muffins, etc. I even adopted a daily habit of snacking on Bit-O-Honey candies. Then one day I made the mistake of watching an episode of *Oprah's Favorite Things*. It was Oprah who introduced me to frozen buttermilk biscuits.

Every Sunday as a child, my family would have homemade biscuits for breakfast. I remember when my father taught me how to make them and how happy the whole family was when that basket of oven fresh fluffy goodness hit the breakfast table. Ah, I can smell them now.

But my love for biscuits was never really about the actual food itself. It was the feelings I experienced while eating them that was the draw. So when Oprah let her secret out the bag and I realized I could have labor-free mouth watering biscuits in 25-30 minutes…I was hooked. I ate them when I was stressed, depressed, too tired to cook but mainly when I wanted to experience some of that happiness from my childhood memory.

Well, the moral of this story is that the biscuits didn't make me happy but they did give me muffin top. And what little nutrients I did have in my body were being used up in the process to break down all that enriched white flour, refined sugar and saturated fat (Oh, did I forget to mention that I was smothering my biscuits in butter and syrup?!). During that time, I became severely nutrient deficient and had no idea. It wasn't until I got educated and starting *eating with a purpose* that my life changed forever.

Eating with a purpose is about giving your body exactly what it needs. Remember when I mentioned earlier that we are constantly regenerating new cells to form new skin, hair, muscle and other important tissues. If you give these cells an ongoing supply of the nutrients that they need to grow and function properly, then the whole body flourishes. Dull hair becomes shiny, dry skin becomes supple, arthritic joints become pain free, blood flows freely through unclogged arteries and so on. It really is that simple.

You've already learned the first step for putting the brakes on aging, which is to avoid those things that destroy our life energy source. Now that we've covered the issue of defense, the second step is to strengthen our offense. We do that by eating with a purpose and choosing foods that meet our body's needs.

What you need to understand is that as we physically age, the body becomes less efficient at absorbing nutrients from food. So when you do the math:

poor diet + age = minimal amounts of nutrients

The goal then is to consume foods that are "nutrient dense" or rich with nutritional content. Not only will this increase nutrient intake but in the long run it can improve the processes of digestion and absorption, no matter how old we are.

This next section will focus on several specific categories of nutrients that play a crucial role in our effort to live long and look good doing it. I will explain why these particular nutrients are important and then identify which foods they can be found in. Be sure to bookmark this section as it will make for a great reference when going grocery shopping or creating new healthy recipes.

ANTIOXIDANTS

Oxidants are the byproducts of the many biological processes that occur within us on a daily basis. Earlier we discussed free radicals, which are a type of oxidant, and talked about how these free radicals cause damage to other cells. Oxidants can also be produced as a result of stress, poor diet, illness and exposure to environmental toxins.

The term *oxidative stress* is used when we have a high quantity of these oxidants in our bodies. In order to combat this condition, nature has provided us with the perfect superhero: antioxidants. Antioxidants are these amazing chemical compounds that have the unique ability of being able to attach themselves to harmful oxidants and neutralize them. So when the body is in a state of oxidative stress, we can prevent cell damage (thereby warding off illness, disease, accelerated aging) by consuming foods that contain potent antioxidant compounds. Below is a list of the most common and most accessible antioxidants and their food sources.

Antioxidant	Function	Signs of Deficiency	Food Sources
Vitamin A	helps to protect against infection and will help strengthen your immune system	acne, dry skin, poor vision, dandruff, and frequent colds	found in beef liver, carrots, cabbage, sweet potatoes, mangos, tomatoes, broccoli and tangerines
Vitamin C	a water soluble nutrient that is great at neutralizing free radicals	bleeding or tender gums, easy bruising, slow wound healing, red pimples on the skin, frequent colds and infections	found in bell peppers, tomato, cabbage, broccoli, cauliflower, strawberries, lemons, kiwi, oranges, grapefruits, and limes
Vitamin E	A fat soluble vitamin that helps the body to use oxygen, form red blood cells, and neutralizes free radicals in the body	easy bruising, slow wound healing, lack of sex drive, infertility, varicose veins	found in wheat germ oil, nuts, sunflower seeds, sesame seeds, tuna, salmon and sweet potatoes
CoenzymeQ 10	fat soluble antioxidant made in the body; critical for good heart health, maintaining energy and blood pressure	poor immune function, and heart disease	found in organ meats, sardines, mackerel, soybean oil, spinach, and peanuts

Selenium	this mineral's antioxidant properties help to protect against free radicals and carcinogens; supports the immune system, and is vital to a healthy male reproductive system	signs of premature aging, cataracts, high blood pressure, frequent infections, family history of cancer	found in tuna, oysters, cottage cheese, cabbage, beef liver, and cod
Carotenoid	natural pigment in fruits and veggies that help to protect against heart disease and helps to lower the risk of certain types of cancer such as prostate and breast cancer		found in brightly colored red, green, yellow and orange fruits and vegetables
Bioflavonoid	natural pigment in fruits and veggies that acts as a powerful antioxidant; also known for anti-inflammatory, anti-cancer and anti-allergen properties	Easy bruising, varicose veins, frequent sprains	found in fruits and veggies that are blue, purple, and deep red in color *also found in dark chocolate

B VITAMINS

B Vitamins are water soluble nutrients that depend on each other's presence in the body in order to be most effective; in other words, they all work together. They are vital to maintaining a healthy nervous system, combating stress, balancing hormones, producing healthy red blood cells and producing/protecting our DNA. The following chart will help you to decide which B vitamins you may be deficient in and which foods you can eat to replenish these nutrients.

Vitamin	Function	Signs of Deficiency	Food Sources
B1 Thiamine	enhances brain function and helps body utilize protein	tender muscles, eye pains, poor concentration, poor memory, prickly legs, tingling hands	watercress, squash, zucchini, asparagus, peas, beans mushroom
B2 Riboflavin	converts fats, sugar, and protein into energy; needed to repair and maintain healthy skin, nails, and eyes	burning eyes, sensitivity to light, sore tongue, cataracts, eczema, split nails, cracked lips	watercress, cabbage, asparagus, broccoli, pumpkin, milk, wheat germ
B3 Niacin	Balances blood sugar, lower cholesterol and aids in energy production	low energy, depression, anxiety, tender or bleeding gums, diarrhea	tuna, chicken, salmon, asparagus, turkey

B5 **Pantothenic** **Acid**	aids in energy production, controls fat metabolism, helps make anti-stress hormones, needed for hair and skin maintenance	muscle tremors or cramps, poor concentration, lack of energy, anxiety or tension, tender heels	avocados, lentils, peas, alfalfa sprouts, eggs, whole wheat
B6 **Pyridoxine**	essential for protein digestion, brain function, and hormone production; natural antidepressant	water retention, tingling hands, depression, irritability, muscle tremors, lack of energy, flaky skin	bananas, brewer's yeast, brown rice, carrots, chicken, eggs, fish
B9 **Folic Acid**	critical for brain development and overall nervous system health	anemia, cracked lips, eczema, premature gray hair, anxiety, poor appetite, stomach pain, depression	leafy greens, liver, wheat germ, spinach, peanuts, sprouts, broccoli, sesame seeds
B12	needed for utilizing protein and blood formation; needed for synthesis of DNA	poor hair condition, dermatitis, irritability, pale skin, constipation, sore muscles	Oysters, sardines, clams, crab, fish, eggs, turkey, chicken

Biotin	promotes healthy skin, nails, and hair	dry skin, dry hair, premature gray hair, poor appetite, dermatitis, tender or sore muscles	oysters, cauliflower, tomatoes, grapefruit, eggs, watermelon, sweet corn, almonds, herring

GARLIC

It keeps away vampires and has the ability to decrease your risk of heart disease, lower cholesterol and reduce the risk of stomach and colon cancers. It contains allicin, a substance that has antiviral, antifungal and antibacterial properties. Garlic has been used for thousands of years because of the many sulfur compounds it contains, giving it great healing potential. These compounds are released when garlic is pressed, crushed, minced and then consumed, whether raw or cooked. Add this odiferous herb to soups, sauces, dressings, rubs, seasonings, spreads, salads and most dishes for a health boost.

SPICES

There are a bounty of herbs and spices that are beneficial to aiding you in your quest for good health and longevity. But there is one specific spice I want to spotlight that is known for its ability to fight off disease. Turmeric, which is also considered an antioxidant, contains phytochemicals that can help normal cells from turning into cancer cells. It is the bright yellow pigment of this popular Indian spice that contains the compound curcumin, which gives it its anti-inflammation properties. A regular diet of this spice can assist you in the prevention of cancer, the reduction of cholesterol levels and lower your risk for blood clot formation.

HEALTHY FATS

The smaller components of healthy fat are referred to as essential fatty acids. They are crucial for slowing the aging process. If you read or listen to health related news, there is no doubt that you've heard the mention of omega-3. This essential fatty acid is making modern science headlines; not because it's new on the scene, but because our diets have become severely deficient. We do not have the necessary enzyme required to produce this fatty acid, therefore we must get it from our food. The problem is that cooking and processing destroys its healthy properties. The deficiency occurs when our diet consists mainly of processed foods that fail to provide us with a good source of essential fatty acids.

Omega-3 is found in cold water fish such as salmon, mackerel, herring, sardines, tuna, and anchovies. Plant sources of omega-3 are pumpkin, flaxseed, walnut, wheat germ and sunflower seed oil. Omega-3 fatty acids play an important role in; infant growth and development, brain development and maintenance, mood stabilization, maintenance of HDL cholesterol, reduction of inflammation, eye health, burn healing, arthritis prevention, production of hormones and male/female reproductive health.

It's important that your diet also include a good balance of omega-3 and omega-6 oils. Omega-6 works together with omega-3 to regulate the body process of inflammation. Omega-6 fatty acids are often used to treat pain associated with arthritis, joint swelling and symptoms of PMS. Two of the best sources are borage oil and evening primrose oil.

By now, you should notice that chapter 3 and chapter 4 of this guide are related to your diet. They specifically outline the two most effective ways in which you can slow the aging process: through protection and dietary intake.

Maintaining good health and a youthful appearance requires that you create new habits for how you treat your body. To help you with that, I want you to take a minute and reflect on what it was like when you were a baby. Remember when your parents fussed over you and did whatever they had to in order to keep you safe? Some of them even read books and sought out advice from others just to make sure they didn't neglect you or cause you any harm. They didn't put soda in your bottle or sprinkle your baby food with salt. They kept you away from harsh chemicals and fed you every few hours. Back then you ate a diet of fruits, vegetables, and whole grains and not only did you like it but you thrived! Your skin was soft and radiant and your hair glistened in the sun. Everything you ate came right back out, albeit more frequently than your parents would have liked.

Most important is that you were healthy and grew into the adult that you are now. What I'm trying to get you to see is that we had it right when we were babies. The lifestyle that I'm suggesting to you isn't something new. You've done it before. It's about getting back to the basics and "babying" yourself. Treat your body as the precious, invaluable gift that it has always been. Protect it from the things that can harm it and feed it the foods that will nourish it and keep it young and healthy.

Chapter 5: The Fountain of Youth

According to Steve Meyerowitz, author of *Water – The Ultimate Cure*, the average adult contains 10 to 13 gallons of water: our blood is 83% water, muscles 75%, brain 75%, heart 75%, bones 22% and our lungs are 86% water! Here is a list of some of the important functions in the human body that involves the use of water.

1. Delivers oxygen to the cells
2. Transports nutrients
3. Hydrates cells
4. Carry electrical charges to other cells
5. Flushes toxins
6. Removes waste
7. Lubricates joints
8. Acts as shock absorber for joints/organs
9. Regulates body temperature
10. Promotes natural healing process

Fairly impressive isn't it? Yet, we don't seem to give water the bragging rights that it deserves. Many people know that a body with no water would die in a matter of days, but there are still some people who go an entire day without drinking any. The truth is that many people are walking around dehydrated and don't even know it. They may feel fatigued, irritable and have a headache and credit it all to a bad day at work when in fact, they are probably thirsty.

> *Dr. Batmanghelidj, one of the world's leading hydration crusaders, suggest that the majority of modern ailments are the result of poor hydration, "Chronic cellular dehydration of the body is the primary etiology of painful, degenerative disease."*

So it only makes sense that the next thing on our list of "ways to stay young" (and alive!) is water consumption.

It's no coincidence that movies and books have always depicted the elusive and mystical Fountain of Youth as a glistening pool of water. Take for example the movie *Cocoon*; Wilford Brimley didn't discover a magic pill that turned back the hands of time. For him, the gateway to experiencing eternal youth was through water. In fact, the mythical Fountain of Youth that has been whispered about over thousands of years is nothing more than a spring of pure water. This water was said to be the purest on earth and capable of restoring youth and vigor.

I want to go on record to say that I believe water is one of the most important nutrients in our diet (and it's not just me, even the USDA lists water as a major nutrient). That's because it is instrumental in two vital body processes that can stop accelerated aging: detoxification and hydration.

People often associate detoxification with alcohol or substance abuse treatment. The theory being that when you abuse alcohol and drugs, the accumulation of these substances creates a condition of toxicity. Well, the very same thing happens when we eat foods laden with chemicals and expose ourselves to harmful elements in the environment. We become toxic.

During my time working as a drug counselor, I was a witness to the body's amazing ability to recover, even after years and years of abuse. Some patients came in looking like death warmed over and I often worried that they wouldn't make it through the night. But with consistent care and nourishment, many patients were able to recover and heal. It's important to understand that detoxification is the body's natural inclination to purge poisons and toxins from the body. It can be mild, like in the form of urination or sweating, or violent and painful, like in the instance of vomiting, cramping and diarrhea. Anyone who has ever had food poisoning can relate.

The good news is that you don't have to get food poisoning or go into treatment to rid your body of toxins. I'm going to share with you an inexpensive way to detoxify and flush your system from the comfort of your own home. I mean this is an ancient secret I'm about to share with you so highlight this section or write this down on a Post-It. Ready? Ok, here it goes. You can flush poisons and toxins out of your body by drinking water…lots of it. Did I just blow your mind? No? Well then let me ask you this; if you know what water can do for you, why aren't you drinking more of it? Wait, I think I might know the answer to this one. Based on the responses that I have heard from clients over the years, I'm thinking that it's either because of the bland taste of water or that you don't like having to go to the bathroom all the time. I agree that these are two valid points but let me explain to you why the pros far outweigh the cons.

Let's first address the frequent urination. My only suggestion to you on this matter is to embrace it. When I'm coaching clients to overcome the emotional barriers in their lives that are keeping them from the health and life they want, the first thing I encourage them to do is to change their thought process. If you keep having negative thoughts about how drinking water keeps you in and out of the bathroom all day, then you will continue to not like drinking water.

Change your thoughts about consuming water and you may be surprised to find that it is no longer an issue. For example, I drink between 80 to 90 ounces of water a day, depending on whether or not I have exercised. That's over two liters for you Euros. And this may be too much information for some of you but I make about 7 or 8 trips to the bathroom a day which is only slightly above average. I am not bothered by this because the benefits are greater than the inconvenience.

This is my thought when I drink water; I am helping my body to flush out all the bad stuff. In doing so, I help my digestive tract to eliminate waste and keep regular. I eliminate toxins in my urine rather than through acne on my skin. I hydrate my cells so they function properly. I lubricate my joints so I can do the activities I love without pain, and my skin is not only radiant but youthful. People who walk around with that healthy glow are people who are hydrated. I guarantee you that once you get into the habit and start seeing the benefits, frequent trips to the bathroom will seem like a small price to pay.

Water is thirst-quenching but I know it doesn't always satisfy the taste buds. The issue is that most people are making beverage choices for the purpose of taste and not for health.

The National Health and Nutrition Examination conducted a survey of the average American's food intake which revealed that Americans consume on average, 22.5 teaspoons of added sugar per day with nearly half of those calories coming from soda and fruit juices.

We've already discussed the damaging effects of sugar on the body but I want to make sure you understand the consequences of choosing taste over benefit. When you decide to drink coffee (a diuretic that dehydrates you) or soda (pollutes you with chemicals and empty calories) or even fruit juices (spikes your blood sugar) you essentially kill your desire to drink water. How many times have you finished a large diet Coke and thought to yourself, "Hmm, a glass of water sure sounds good." I'm willing to bet never. For every one serving of these beverages, you deprive your body of a vital nutrient (water) and in the process you destroy other important nutrients like vitamins and minerals.

That's why I'm bewildered by people at restaurants who do contradictory things like eating a healthy spinach salad with balsamic on the side, all while washing it down with several glasses of Coke. That makes as much sense as ordering a veggie burger topped with three strips of bacon.

First of all, try to refrain from drinking anything while eating. A beverage will just dilute your digestive enzymes and inhibit digestion. It's best to drink water 30 minutes before a meal or 30 minutes after. Secondly, when you drink soda or fruit juice, you've just ingested a large quantity of sugar that is going to spike your blood glucose and depending on what you ate; the sugar may sit in your gut and cause fermentation. And by fermentation I mean gas. So by the time you get back to the office, you're already tired, you've compromised the nutrients in your meal, and your noisy gut rumblings are making your coworkers feel uncomfortable. Is it really worth it?

I'm not suggesting that you never drink soda or coffee again, but I am saying that if you must have it, limit it. The majority of your liquid intake should be in the form of water. And keep in mind that beverages like herbal tea, fresh fruit juice (not from concentrate) and fruit itself, contribute to your daily water intake. The goal is to try and consume half of your body weight in ounces. For instance, if you weigh 150 lbs, you should be drinking 75 ounces of water. If you get sick or exercise, then you need to increase this amount. Be sure that its quality water and not just cleverly packaged tap water. I try to avoid bottled water by using a home distiller. Either filter your water with a good charcoal filtration system or research your best bottled options.

Chapter 6: Diagnostic Care

Everyone knows what happens to a car if you don't put fuel in it. It will die on you. It's also important to have regular maintenance on your vehicle to ensure that it keeps running smoothly. That means regular oil changes, replacing filters, rotating tires and, well, you get the picture. The same is true of the human body. Like most cars, we have a built in "maintenance required" notification system that should not be ignored. In chapters 2 and 3, we talked about many of the signs and symptoms you may experience when the body is nutrient deprived or dehydrated. Those signs can also be indicators of a more serious condition or illness manifesting itself inside of your body. The best way to figure out what's going on is with diagnostic care.

This is where I encourage you to utilize access to conventional medicine. The goal is to use the tools of conventional medicine, like testing, as preventative care rather than using it for after care or when a disease has already manifested. Basically, you want to go in for routine maintenance in order to keep from breaking down on your commute through life. To do that, you need to develop a diagnostic care regimen that involves you seeing a physician for annual routine exams.

Now these exams are not going to be like those you've had in the past. You know the kind where you go in, wait an hour only to see the doctor for 15 minutes. He listens to your heart, checks your vitals and weight and then sends you on your way. Those types of visits are a thing of the past. From this moment on, you are a health advocate. Information and knowledge is empowering and it puts you in the position of demanding a higher level of care.

I can recall what it was like sitting in that freezing cold exam room in a paper gown, waiting and thinking of all the things I wanted to ask my doctor. Then he would come in all rushed, barely making eye contact, and before I knew it, he was out the door. I was too intimidated to ask questions and felt like I shouldn't bother such a busy important man. Can you relate?

Once I educated myself and experienced what a real doctor/patient relationship should be like, I felt empowered and began to demand a higher level of care. And a great way to identify the good doctors from the bad ones is in how they react to your personal advocacy. If they refuse you and tell you that your requests are unnecessary, then you know you have a dud. But if they respond to you in a way that makes you feel heard and agree to work collaboratively with you in the prevention of disease, then you have a keeper.

Rest assured that none of the things that I am about to suggest to you are outlandish, invasive or expensive. Cost will depend on the type of insurance you have but for the most part, you should incur minor cost under standard coverage policies.

Note that all of these tests/screens are equally important and should be done on an annual basis. If you are presenting with symptoms of an underlying condition, then some tests will need to be performed on a more frequent basis. These tests/screens are to help you gauge what your body needs and to prevent degenerative disease. The results will also be good indicators as to your current level of health.

Blood Test

Test Type	Purpose
CBC and Differential	This a basic test to determine your blood count
Renal Panel	This screen is to check levels of key minerals, metabolic waste products and kidney function
Liver Panel	A screen to check liver function by measuring enzymes
Blood Glucose	This test requires a period of fasting and gives an accurate assessment of your blood sugar level
C-reactive Protein	A screen/indicator for inflammation in arteries
25-Hydroxy-Vitamin D	This will assess your level of vitamin D; low levels of this vital nutrient can be a precursor for serious health conditions
Lipid Panel	A test to determine cholesterol levels

Urine Sample

A screen of your urine should be completed to test for content of sugar, proteins and the presence of blood

Hair Mineral Analysis

An excellent method of determining the levels of calcium, magnesium, zinc, chromium, selenium, and manganese in the body as well as giving useful information about levels of potentially toxic minerals like aluminum, copper, arsenic and cadmium

Serum Homocysteine

Probably the most important test and best indicator of your current health; the results of this test can help to determine if you are getting sufficient amounts of B vitamins in your diet and is a good indicator of your risk level for heart disease

Pap Smear/Prostate Exam(PSA)

Ladies – I know it is an awkward and somewhat invasive procedure but it is absolutely necessary for maintaining good reproductive health; regular pap smears are the best prevention for cervical cancer and should always be accompanied by a breast exam to screen for lumps or growths

Gents – the same goes for you, I know you'd much rather take a shot to the groin then undergo this exam but if you haven't heard, prostate cancer is on the rise mostly due to a lack of early detection; ignorance is not bliss and it can significantly affect the quality of your life

If you have problems convincing your doctor to perform this type of routine diagnostic care then I have two suggestions for you. 1) Find another doctor who will or 2) Find yourself a holistic health practitioner or naturopathic physician who understands what you are trying to do and respects your intentions to live a long healthy life.

I recommend having these tests done through your insurance and then taking your results to somebody who knows how to interpret them and guide you. If you have low levels of vital minerals and your homocysteine level is high, a conventional medicine man may give you a prescription for a multivitamin and send you on your way. A nutrition specialist or naturopathic physician can help you to determine why you are deficient and identify ways to boost specific nutrient intake. You do not have to settle for subpar care. I repeat…you do not have to settle for subpar care! I want you to start believing that your body deserves the best care possible.

Chapter 7: Move It or Lose It

As we age, our focus tends to shift from being concerned about how our bodies look to being more worried about how our bodies function. We seem to accept daily aches and pains as inevitable or bloated bellies as a natural side effect of aging. We lose all hope of retaining any youthful qualities in our physical appearance and focus solely on making sure our hips won't pop out of joint from a wrong step.

Maybe that's how you used to think before you started reading this book but things have changed. A future of hospitals, medications and inactivity are no longer on the horizon. You envision a life of leisure, independence, vitality and longevity. You recognize that your body is your single most important investment in life and you plan on getting great returns. And this next step has a huge payoff in health benefits.

Before we get into the benefits, let's talk about movement. This secret is aptly titled "move it or lose it" because those are the only two choices when it comes to the health of your body's structure. Our infrastructure (e.g. bones, muscles, ligaments) is what keeps us upright and moving. When we don't maintain this structure, it begins to degenerate.

It is a well known fact that we lose bone density and muscle as we age. It is also well-known that you can prevent this from happening by committing to a lifestyle of movement. I say movement because it is the very act of moving the body that promotes health. We know that our ancestors did not have gyms. People worked all day in the fields and the factories and had no reason to stop off at 24 Hr. Fitness on their way home. The amount and types of movements required to perform their jobs or daily activities was all their bodies needed.

You may not have noticed, but we have become a sedentary generation. We have equipment to farm for us, cars to transport us, and technological advances that have nearly eliminated the need for us to get out of our chairs. Think about it. If you set up a mini fridge right by your filing cabinet in your office, you could swivel your whole day away at your desk.

In 2000, the Journal of Applied Physiology noted a strong correlation between the emergence of modern chronic disease and increased physical inactivity. It reported that approximately 250,000 deaths per year in the US were premature due to physical inactivity.

We pay a price for all of these modern day luxuries and advances: stagnation, obesity, chronic pain, chronic disease and vitamin D deficiency (sunlight has a difficult time finding its way into office buildings). The problem is that when we adapted to this new lifestyle, we forgot about the importance of movement. So if you want to continue to do all the physical activities that you enjoy, you must make movement a regular part of your daily life. Please note that I said daily which I'm sure has some of you questioning, "I haven't exercised in years; does she expect me to work out every day?" Well the answer is I don't and let me explain why.

There are varying degrees of movement, but the two that we are going to pay particular interest in are exercise and physical activity. Exercise includes those aerobic activities that are going to increase your heart rate, increase your endurance and build muscle. Physical activity includes those routine activities that you perform throughout the day that promote balance, strength, flexibility and endurance. It is the addition of these two forms of movement into your lifestyle that is going to improve your health and appearance and reduce your risk of injury and disease.

One thing that conventional medicine and alternative medicine agree on is the importance of cardiovascular and aerobic exercise. Some of the health benefits include:

- *Reduced risk of hypertension, heart disease and diabetes*

- *Weight control and caloric balance*

- *Reduced risk of disability and/or injury*

- *Improved balance and flexibility*

- *Improved disposition and mood*

Unfortunately, many people struggle with the commitment of regular exercise. I personally believe it is because they may have set unrealistic goals for themselves or they continue to hold the desire of wanting immediate results. According to *Medical News Today*, 80% of gym memberships go unused. It's a twofold problem of people losing motivation and new members having poor instruction or no guidance at all. In my health coaching business, I approach this challenge by addressing three factors: my client's current level of fitness; their interest and goals; and their willingness to invest and learn.

Say, for example, you are my client and want to start an exercise program. First I would assess your level of physical fitness. Do you already workout? Was the last show you worked out to Jack LaLane or Tony Horton's *P90X*? Next, I want to know if you have a specific goal in mind or just want to improve your overall fitness level. An important part of this assessment is determining what type of exercise you enjoy. Starting a workout program that is based on exercises you hate will only set you up to fail. Do you hate to run but love biking? Would you prefer to use resistance bands because you feel awkward working with free weights? The goal is to create a regimen that offers variety and includes things you like (or at least can tolerate) so you don't get bored.

The last thing I assess with my clients is how much work they are willing to put into it. That's because getting fit involves discipline and getting educated. For this to work, you either need to enlist the help of a professional or learn it on your own. Setting up this program does not have to be expensive or overwhelming. In fact, I am going to give you some tips on how to make it easier on yourself.

Tip 1 - If you can afford it, get a qualified personal trainer; preferably one that will come to your home and show you how to properly exercise with few, if any props. A great trainer will show you how to use household items or inexpensive equipment to assist in your workouts. Tell them that you will retain them for a predetermined amount of time (depends on how much you want to spend and your learning curve) and that you want them to teach you how to properly exercise on your own. You don't need a trainer for the rest of your life...just long enough to get you on your way.

Tip 2 - If you can't afford a trainer, teach yourself. There is an endless supply of books, DVD's, and online tutorials that can help you. I typically recommend my fit clients to do an maintaining target heart rate) AND two days of strength training. For those clients that have been inactive, I suggest starting with one hour of daily physical activity and strength training twice a week; then a gradual increase to performing aerobic exercise.

If you are reading carefully, you'll notice that I recommend strength training for everyone, regardless of level of fitness. This does not mean that I have all my clients in the gym bench pressing, but I do encourage them all to do some form of weight resistance.

What I'm about to say is very important to those of us on the other side of forty, so pay close attention. We must build muscle to strengthen our core, to strengthen our infrastructure, and to prevent conditions such as arthritis and joint pain. And if that doesn't convince you, take note that muscle burns fat. You are more likely to burn fat by building muscle than by cardio alone. More muscle increases your metabolism, the rate at which you burn calories.

But wait, it gets better! Done properly, strength training can also be a cardio workout in the form of interval training. You can raise your target heart rate and build muscle all at the same time. I highly recommend the "super slow technique" by

Ken Hutchins. It is a great technique that produces amazing results while reducing risk of injury because it is performed with very controlled movements. This is a perfect option for older adults.

Tip 3 - Get a gym membership but on your terms. Working out at a gym works well for some people but don't get pressured into it. If you go in knowing exactly what you want, chances are you leave feeling happy with your purchase and more likely to return. Here are some suggestions to help you get the best deal.

Find a gym that gives you a discounted membership for restricted days. For example, instead of paying for 7 days a week when you're only going 2-3 times per week, opt to get a membership that restricts your usage to certain days of the week. This actually helps you to stick to a regimen because there are only so many days per week that you can use the facility. You can save yourself as much as $10 -$20 a month.

Forgo the bells and whistles. Do you really need access to racquetball courts or a juice bar? All you need are cardio machines, free weights and weight machines. For swimmers, find a gym with a pool so you can swim year round.

If you want to save some money and think the gym feels more like a social gathering, then you are much better off getting a membership at your local community center. They tend to be cheaper, let you go month to month and are less crowded.

Tip 4 - If you truly hate the idea of going to the gym then don't waste your money on a membership. Instead, sign up for classes at a community center or community college. Start a walking or running group with friends or join a fitness group on social networking sites like Meetup.com.

Tip 5 - If you like to work out at home, invest in exercise DVD's or online programs. Do your kids or grandkids have an Xbox or Playstation you can use? There are some excellent workout programs for adults on these consoles like The Biggest Loser workout for Xbox.

The best advice I can give you when it comes to exercise is to be realistic in setting your goals. It will take some time before you see the rewards so don't get discouraged. The expectation is that you perform some type of exercise two times per week if you've been inactive and four times a week if you experience some level of fitness.

For those who have medical issues that impair their abilities or if you have not been cleared by your physician to perform physical exercise, I recommend that you at least engage in some type of physical activity on a daily basis. Physical activity is anything that makes your body move at a pace that requires you to exert energy, e.g., dancing, mowing the lawn, gardening, playing with children, cleaning the garage, washing the car, washing the dog, or walking the dog. Performing regular acts of bending, kneeling, pulling, reaching, stepping, turning, and squatting promote balance and flexibility. Try to do about thirty minutes of physical activity outside in the sun to promote the synthesis of Vitamin D.

As a holistic health coach, I am a staunch advocate for body work which includes activities such as yoga and Tai Chi. These exercises focus on controlled movements and breathing techniques which are immensely beneficial to circulation, concentration, coordination, and memory. It also is an excellent way to increase oxygen intake and learn correct methods of breathing. More importantly, it helps to create a balance between the mind and body so that you become more aware of what your body needs.

To help you understand the importance behind the "move it or lose it" theory, I want you to conduct a little experiment. The next time you are at your doctor's office or at the hospital visiting someone, take a look around you. Look at the doctors, the nurses, the office staff and especially the patients. Chances are, at least half of the people there are overweight or out of shape. They probably live sedentary lives, rely on medications or have relinquished control of their health and put it in the hands of doctors and insurance providers. There is something not quite right when a doctor is on the same high blood pressure medication as his patients. That's like having a dentist with really bad teeth.

Next, go and visit a yoga studio or gym or a wellness center. Chances are that you will see very few people who are overweight and out of shape. These individuals are the ones who have taken responsibility for their own health. Every day that they show up, they are investing in their future. They don't think of getting old; they think of living well. This is where you want to spend your time…in the company of people who are where you want to be. Every time you find yourself making excuses for not being physically active, I want you to stop and visualize what it would be like to live in an assisted care facility, totally dependent on some burly tattooed man who makes $10.25 an hour to take care of you. Enough said.

Chapter 8: Supporting Your Immune System

Imagine for a moment that you are the manager of a talented up-and-coming athlete. This young athlete is dependent on you to make decisions in regard to the longevity and success of his career. The game plan is to allow this talented young man the opportunity to develop his skills and learn the important techniques and strategies that will eventually help him to be a strong competitor.

Over the next several years, he will experience many matches and be exposed to different types of conditions but in the long run, you know the consistent training will pay off with a championship. But then you are approached by a trainer that tells you he can arrange for your athlete to compete against the current champion in one month. He says that he will provide special training for your guy to get him prepared for the fight. You know that your guy is talented and that the trainer is the best in the business and you are excited at the thought of him becoming a champion in just one month. You also recognize that your guy could get hurt or seriously injured due to his lack of experience. So, what do you do?

I ask because although you may not be the manager of a talented athlete, you are the manager of your body. The truth is that you face a similar decision making process every time your body is put in the situation of having to fight: whether it's fighting a cold or battling cancer.

When your health is being jeopardized by infection or disease, you are required to make a decision in regard to how you will go about fighting. And the talented athlete that you manage in real life is your immune system. It is amazing. It is fighting for you when you are sick and protecting you when you are well.

The question is what kind of manager are you? Do you take care of you immune system by giving it the things it needs to get stronger and letting it do so on its own natural schedule. Or do you call on your immune system to do battle for you without giving it what it needs to be strong, thereby putting it at risk of harm? No one wants a long drawn out battle but trying to get rid of symptoms with quick fixes like antibiotics and steroids often cause collateral damage.

I won't bore you with the intricate details of how the immune system works and frankly there is still a bit of mystery to this magnificent regulatory system. It is important though to understand the basics. Your immune system is responsible for surveying, identifying, responding, and adjusting to foreign invasions by microorganisms.

The Lymphatic system is at the core of our immune system and acts as the transportation highway for white blood cells to get to areas of infection, injury or abnormal cell growth. Every time your immune system locates a microorganisms, it goes through the process of identifying it, determining how to best combat it, and then committing to memory the battle plans in case of any future invasions.

What we want to pay close attention to are those things that will weaken or destroy the immune system and those nutrients, herbs, and behaviors that will strengthen it. In our quest to slow down the aging of our cells, it is imperative that we build up a strong defense which equates to having a healthy immune system.

Let us first look at those things that pose a threat to our immune system.

THREATS

Alcohol	excessive use can impair your immune system's ability to function; it weakens the central nervous system and depletes many of the vitamins and minerals (e.g. folic acid, vitamin E, magnesium, zinc) that are crucial to good immune health
Aspartame	this artificial sweetener breaks down into a toxic substance in the digestive tract and destroys nutrients; suppresses the immune system by impairing lymphocyte activity

Caffeine	compounds in this substance suppress immune functions
Sodium Nitrate	preservative found in cured meats; can damage the central nervous system
Antibiotics	known immune system suppressor; destroys healthy bacteria in the gut and allows for harmful particles to be absorbed into the bloodstream
Meat	the high protein content of meat depletes calcium in the body and is a source of antibiotics and hormones
Heavy Metals	metals such as cadmium, lead and mercury are toxic to the body and depress cells of the lymphatic system
Stress	especially prolonged periods of stress can wreak havoc on the immune system by creating free radicals and depleting nutrients; stress can impair thymus gland functioning and depresses lymphocyte production

The good news is that if you have already enacted the practices discussed in previous chapters of this guidebook, you are well on your way to strengthening your immune system. Avoiding toxins, eliminating junk foods, and eating a diet rich in nutrients and antioxidants are key components to promoting healthy immunity.

Exercise and getting adequate amounts of sleep are equally important. Adding the following supplements to your diet can also help to support your immune system.

Dietary Supplements	Why you may need it
A good quality multivitamin	as we age our ability to absorb nutrients decreases so it is often necessary to supplement our diet with a multivitamin and multi-mineral; this is especially true for people who have diets high in sugar and processed foods
Vitamin C	most multivitamins don't have adequate dosage of this vitamin so take an additional supplement of 1,000 grams three times a day
Echinacea	an herb that can be taken in tea or capsule form; helps to stimulate activity of immune cells (consult with an integrative healthcare provider if you have allergies or are on medications; do not use if you have an autoimmune disease)
Astragalus	an herb that has antiviral properties and enhances immune cell activity (consult with an integrative healthcare provider if you have diabetes or are on anti-coagulant medications; do not use if you have a fever)

Probiotic	*these beneficial bacteria will help to promote a healthy digestive tract and limit disease causing bacteria*
Garlic	*has antimicrobial and antiviral properties and if consumed regularly, can protect against infection*

Having a strong immune system can be the difference between having an upset stomach and having the stomach flu. It also makes the difference between having energy and rarely getting sick versus having chronic fatigue and chronic illness. Just keep in mind that you are responsible for managing the health of your immune system. Are you going to send it into battle unprepared to fight or are you going to support it in being the ultimate fighting champion that it's intended to be?

Chapter 9: Relax, Rest and Repair

At last, we have made it our final destination in our journey to rediscover our youth. This next step won't cost you any money and if done religiously, can maybe even add years to your life. It is the dependent relationship of these three factors that is the foundation of creating a balance between your mind and your body. When your mind and body are out of sync, you become vulnerable to disease, aging, mood disorders, cognitive disorders and toxicity. When the two are balanced and in alignment with one another, you can achieve peace, vitality, optimal health and clarity.

It's just like when your modem and your computer are not properly connected: your computer cannot perform at its full potential. So in order to facilitate a connectedness between your mind and body, three things must occur: relaxation, rest, and repair.

According to a 2007 study by the American Psychological Association, approximately 75 to 90 percent of all doctor office visits are for stress-related ailments and complaints. Nearly half of participants in this study reported that their stress level had increased over the past five years and that they have either over eaten or eaten unhealthy foods due to stress.

Stress is a part of life and it would be unrealistic for me to suggest that you can eliminate it all together. During my years of working with families and clients battling serious health problems, I often suggested to them to reduce the stress in their lives. It wasn't until my own personal physician said the same thing to me ten years ago that I realized how asinine it sounded.

What if the major stress in your life was your job, or the care of your special needs child, or your living arrangement? What do you do when quitting or moving is not an option? So I changed the way that I encouraged my clients to deal with stress. Now I say "You need to reduce your stress in the areas of your life that you can, and learn to manage your stress in those areas of your life where it is unavoidable."

In chapter three, we discussed how the body responds to stress and the toll that it takes on your health. Now we need to focus on what we can do to either reduce stress or manage it.

Reducing stress may be difficult for some because it involves letting go of outcomes or relinquishing control of the things that are beyond our control (e.g., cancelled flights or traffic). Your response to a physical, mental, social or emotional stimulus is what initiates stress. It's actually not the event itself but how we react to it. In order to reduce stress in your life, you have to make a conscious effort to not respond negatively or remove the stimuli altogether.

For example, you can choose not to internalize someone's anger and let them own it, or accept that you are late for an appointment and recognize that it is not worth getting into an accident over. In the case of removing a stimulus, you may have to end a stressful relationship, learn to say no without the guilt, or stop watching the news/reading the paper. Take back control of your thoughts and don't spend time worrying about something that has yet to happen or that can't be fixed. Here are two of my favorite quotes that serve as great reminders of how pointless it is to worry about the future.

"Worry never robs tomorrow of its sorrow, it only saps today of its joy." ~ *Leo Buscaglia*

"Troubles are a lot like people—they grow bigger if you nurse them." ~ *Unknown Author*

Managing the everyday stressors in our lives that are unavoidable requires that we become more aware of our habit of thinking. Emotional (mental) stress is when we have prolonged thoughts that invoke feelings of fear, worry and anxiety; whereas physical stress is when our body is subjected to a prolonged state of physical excitement, tension or pain (stimulus).

The key to managing stress is to recognize when you are experiencing a period of prolonged physical or emotional stress. I know it sounds as if I may have simplified the condition but that is exactly what it boils down to. Your body is capable of dealing with the "flight or fight" syndrome in small spurts. But it's the prolonged periods of stress that are killing us.

I use to love haunted houses as a kid. Actually, I still do. What a thrill to slowly creep through a dark hallway; frightened and excited all at the same time, never quite knowing what was going to happen. My heart would race, and my whole body felt like it was in a heightened state of anticipation! I never wanted that feeling to end but thank goodness it did. Can you imagine walking around all day in a heightened state like that? Well, that is exactly what we do when we carry stress with us. It is physically and emotionally taxing on our bodies. But if you are able to stop and recognize that you are having compulsive thoughts or that you have been walking around with a clenched jaw for the past two hours, you give yourself an opportunity to abort that state of mind.

When you focus on stressors, it's like stoking a fire. It will only make it grow. When you take the focus off of the stressors, the feelings associated with the stress will diminish or extinguish all together. Feelings are like gears in a car, we can switch them at any time or even change directions if we want. I have found that the best way to initiate this change in thinking or focus is to engage in an activity that you like or something that requires your full attention. A few examples would be: exercise, physical activity, watching sports highlights, singing, dancing, playing with a child, playing with your dog, looking at old photos, or watching a comedy.

If you are stressed out at work, take a minute to call a friend who always makes you laugh. If you have been carrying stress in your body (e.g., tense shoulders, clenched jaw, furrowed brows, tightness in your chest), alleviate it by engaging in activities that help you to relax like reading or taking a hot bath. Just a few minutes are enough to actually stop the release of stress hormones and lower your blood pressure.

Meditation, yoga, Tai Chi, massage, deep breathing, a nap and connecting with nature are also good ways to shift your thoughts and return the body to a state of balance. For long-term reduction of stress, look at improving your time management skills, learn to say no, and set realistic expectations for yourself and others.

If you experience a high level of stress in your life, you may benefit from taking a supplement to help you manage. In addition to the B vitamins, CoQ10, calcium and magnesium that you should already be taking, try adding Inositol which can help stabilize moods. I also suggest taking a supplement that contains a Theanine (200mg) and GABA (200 – 500 mg) combination that has significant calming effects on the brain. I personally drink a variety of herbal teas that act as gentle relaxants. At the end of a long stressful day, try drinking a cup of chamomile, passionflower, kava kava or St. John's Wort. These teas will also help you to get a good night's sleep.

Speaking of which, sleeping is the next element I want to discuss in our mission of creating mind/body balance. If you have trouble relaxing, then chances are that you also have problems sleeping. Again, these two elements are totally dependent on each other so it's crucial for you to master the art of relaxation. Sleep is essential for proper immune function and for restoring the body both physically and mentally. But we're not talking just any kind of sleep. When I tell you that you need to get a good night's sleep, I am referring to that deep, restorative (referred to as delta sleep or non-REM) sleep that unfortunately shortens in duration as we get older.

A good balance of REM (Rapid Eye Movement) and non-REM sleep allows for the body to regenerate and repair. You may not think much is going on when you're asleep but your body is actually hard at work with cell division, protein synthesis, muscle tissue repair, absorption of nutrients and in preparing the body for elimination.

A chronic lack of sleep or insomnia can cause mood swings, cognitive impairment and has been linked to diseases such as diabetes and heart disease. More importantly, hormone secretion occurs while we sleep and ongoing deprivation seems to cause symptoms of accelerated aging. Think about how much growth and development occurs in children. No wonder they need up to 10 to 12 hours a night! The goal for you is to strive to get at least seven to eight hours each night. And avoid those things that can reduce your chances of a good night's sleep, such as having the TV on in the background, working in bed, drinking caffeine and alcohol near bedtime, or eating late night sugary snacks.

Daily Guide to Health and Wellness

I know what you're thinking—this sounds like a lot of work! And to some degree, you are right. Changing the health and condition of your body is going to require effort on your part. This is not a crash diet or a quick fix gimmick to losing weight. This is about making a decision and commitment to caring for your body in a way that allows you to live free from medical intervention. It's also about wanting to look youthful and live a life that is free of pain and illness.

You no longer buy into the belief that getting older means your body will fall apart and that you must willingly accept this as your fate. You've wised up to the fact that the food, drug, and healthcare industries profit off of your poor health and you refuse to be their sucker. Most importantly, you understand that incorporating the *Secrets to Healthy Aging* into your lifestyle will be easier and cheaper than battling a life threatening disease. You just have to choose between working to stay healthy or working to do damage repair.

If you are like me and want to make this one life the best it can possibly be, then you are going to have to start taking better care of yourself. And I promise you that once you start to feel and see the benefits, it will make all the effort worthwhile. If you incorporate *The Secrets to Healthy Aging* into your daily routine, it will make all the difference. And soon it will stop feeling like work and will just become a part of your lifestyle.

Now that you have finished this guidebook, you know exactly what to do. But just to help you along, I've created this cheat sheet that you can use as a reference to guide you through the day. Each morning, I want you to review the cheat sheet and implement each practice into your day. And if you prefer 1 on 1 coaching to help get you started, don't hesitate to contact me at:

info@CoachNikole.com

I'm so proud of you for taking back control of your health; know with certainty that you are on your way to looking and feeling your best...for life!

Keeping You Informed & Keeping You Well,

~Coach Nikole

Daily Health Cheat Sheet

Avoid harmful chemicals and toxic substances

Limit my alcohol, caffiene and sugar intake

Drink enough water to = 1/2 my body weight in ounces

Eat 6-8 servings of brightly colored fruits and vegetables

Engage in 60 minutes of physical activity outside or perform at least 30 minutes of aerobic exercise at my target heart rate

Take an antioxidant supplement or eat three servings of foods that contain antioxidants

Take a multi-vitamin and a multi-mineral

Manage my stress by shifting my thoughts and having realistic expectations of myself and others

Get 7-8 Hours of sleep tonight

About the Author

Nikole Seals' health coach practice began as a result of her own experience with chronic illness. Her newfound revelations enabled her to transform her life to the extent that, today, she experiences daily optimal health. Her passion for helping others led her to create a series of guidebooks and resource tools to help motivate and educate people on ways to achieve their health goals: whether it's weight loss, healthy aging, or raising healthy kids. She remains firm in her practice of providing consumers with current information and quality products.

Nikole Seals has over twenty years experience working with adults and children, helping them to improve their health and quality of life with proper nutrition and life management coaching. She has worked as a youth counselor, fitness trainer, family therapist, social worker, nutrition counselor, health advocate, and substance abuse counselor. She holds a BS in Human Development and a Master's Degree in Social Work. She is trained as a Holistic Nutritional Consultant and is a member of the National Association of Nutritional Consultants, the National Association of Social Workers, a leader with the Prevent Obesity Network, and a published author of educational guides for international students of social work with Cinahl Information Systems.

Nikole operates Nourished Minds out of Orange County, CA and offers in-person and online services to include coaching, webinars, educational guides, books and motivational speaking.

Connect with Nikole online
For more information about coaching services
visit: CoachNikole.com
Watch Videos, Read Guides, and Get Books &
Programs at:
NourishedMinds.com

Email: info@CoachNikole.com

References

Atkins, R.C. (2000). *Dr. Atkins's age defying diet revolution.* New York: St. Martin's Press.

Balch, P.A. (2006). *Prescription for nutritional healing* (3rd Ed.). New York: Penguin Group.

Bowden, J. (2008). *The most effective natural cures on earth.* Beverly, MA: Fair Winds Press.

Holford, P. (2004). *The new optimum nutrition bible* (Rev. Ed.). Berkeley, CA: Crossing Press.

Meyerowitz, S. (2001). *Water: The ultimate cure.* Summertown, TN: Book Publishing Company.

Somer, E. (2006). *Age proof your body: Your complete guide to looking and feeling younger.* New York: McGraw-Hill.

Tenney, L. (1986). *The immune system: A nutritional approach.* U.S.A.: Woodland Health Books.

Torkos, S. (2010). *Relax.* Better Nutrition Healthy Living guide (15). Better Nutrition. El Segundo, CA: Active Interest Media Inc.

U.S. Census Bureau. (2011). Age and sex composition. (US Census Bureau Publication No. C2010BR-03) http://www.census.gov/prod/cen2010/briefs/c2010br-03.pdf

Warren, J. L., Bacon, W. E., Harris, T., McBean, A. M., Foley, D. J., and Phillips, C. (1994) **The burden and outcomes associated with dehydration among US elderly, 1991.** *American Journal of Public Health*, **84,** 1265 - 1269.

Weil, Andrew. (2011). *You can't afford to get sick: Your guide to Optimum Health and Health Care.* New York: Penguin Group.

Wexler, B. (2007). *Antioxidants: Natural defense against oxidative stress*. Orem, UT: Woodland Publishing.

www.ingramcontent.com/pod-product-compliance
Lightning Source LLC
Chambersburg PA
CBHW050542280326
41933CB00011B/1691